THE BEAUTY OF NATURAL BIRTH CONTROL

A WOMEN'S GUIDE TO FEMALE BARRIER BIRTH CONTROL

JENNIFER ANNE HOLLEY

The information in this book is not intended as medical advice or to replace the medical advice of a licensed health care professional. It is intended to share the personal knowledge, research and experience of the author, Jennifer Anne Holley. The author expressly disclaims any responsibility for any liability, loss or risk, personal or otherwise, which is incurred as a result of using any of the information or recommendations expressed in this book. You are encouraged to make your own health care decisions in partnership with a health care professional. If you have any questions or concerns, please contact the appropriate health care professional.

ISBN-13: 978-0-578-56463-0

TABLE OF CONTENTS

A great and wise man, David Henry Thoreau, once wrote: "What you get by achieving your goals is not as important as what you become by achieving your goals." (Thoreau)

I dedicate this book to my daughter, Kendall. May you touch the world with a loving heart and healing hands.

~M~

JENNIFER ANNE HOLLEY

PREFACE

"A Journey of a Thousand Miles Begins with a Single Step," a quote by Lao-Tzu 4th century BC is the philosophy I used to guide me along my journey. At times it felt as though I walked a thousand miles, but every single step was worth it once I reached my destination. I always dreamed of becoming a doctor or nurse, specializing in female health. Fate led me down another path to realizing my ambition. I spent many years researching and writing this book, and in which I recognized my true calling.

I became a female barrier user when I was in my early thirties, and I have been using caps and diaphragms exclusively ever since. When I first started using caps and diaphragms, I was fortunate enough to come across a group of very supportive and knowledgeable women. It was in the Yahoo Group, DiaphragmsAndCaps, where I learned a lot about this empowering method of birth control. I am thankful to the members and moderators for sharing their experiences with me and for inviting me to be a group moderator. The time I spent working on the advisory board of the discussion group is where I formed my passion for natural birth control. I want to thank all the ladies in the group, for you are indeed an inspiration!

I want to thank all those who supported me in this endeavor, especially my family and friends. Thank you to my husband and children for their love and encouragement, particularly my daughter, for it was in having a daughter of my own that inspired me more than anything to create this guide for women. A special thank you to my dear friend, Carol, who read my work and offered valuable insight. I am sincerely grateful to Dr. Trevor Wing of the Women's Natural Health Clinic, who has spent countless hours reading and editing for me, and to his colleagues who have helped me along the way. You have accompanied me down a long and challenging road, and I couldn't have done it without you! Thank you for believing in me and encouraging me to finish this valuable work.

It is with great enthusiasm that I welcome you into the world of female barrier birth control! I hope the information in my book will serve as an inspiration to you on your quest for natural birth control. I am confident the resources included, as well as my guidance and support, will empower you to a happier, healthier way of life. Please recommend my book to any of your female family members and friends interested in switching to, or starting to use natural, affordable birth control methods.

CHAPTER 1

~

MY JOURNEY

I was eighteen when I decided it was time to go to my first gynecology appointment. At that time, it was recommended that a young woman should have her first Pap smear and gynecology exam when she turned eighteen or when she first became sexually active. In those days, when a woman said she was going to the doctor for birth control what she meant was she was going to the doctor to get on "the pill." When I set up my first appointment; I just assumed I would be prescribed hormonal birth control pills as well.

I asked friends and family for recommendations for a doctor, and ultimately, I decided on a male gynecologist referred to me by a female friend. I went by myself to the appointment, and I felt nervous leading up to it. I arrived at the doctor's office, and there was a waiting room full of people. I signed in, and the receptionist gave me paperwork to fill out and told me to have a seat. Shortly after that, a nurse called me back.

The first part of the appointment was a consultation in the doctor's office. I recall the initial meeting being a very awkward experience. I was not prepared at all for what would happen during the consult nor the physical exam.

I sat in the consultation room, fully dressed, and very nervous. When the doctor arrived, he began asking me what I knew about birth control and which type I wanted to use.

I perceived him as standoffish, and I did not sense any real concern for me as a patient. He talked fast, and the meeting felt rushed. After a very brief discussion, I concluded that "the pill" was the preferred option for all his patients, so that is what I agreed to. The doctor did not offer the choice of a diaphragm or cervical cap at any time during the appointment, nor did he discuss the use of condoms for protection from sexually transmitted infections (STI's) .

The next phase of the appointment took place in the examination room. I observed a table with stirrups covered with a long and narrow paper sheet on it. The nurse handed me a white paper gown cover-up. She told me to undress from the waist down and that the doctor would be in shortly.

I waited for what seemed like an eternity but was, in fact, only a few short minutes. All the while, my anxiety was building. When the doctor entered the room, he performed my first pelvic exam and did a Pap smear. It was not painful, but it was not comfortable either. The speculum felt cold, but it was over fairly quickly. I then got dressed and waited for the nurse to come in with my prescription and instructions. I left that day with a very unsatisfied feeling. My experience at the appointment was unacceptable to me, and it set the stage for my attitude toward future gynecology appointments.

Things did get better for me down the road. I never went for a follow up to that particular gynecologist. I found someone else who was more attuned to the feelings of his patients. It was altogether a better experience, yet I remained on hormonal birth control for many years to come. Knowing what I know now, I look back and see the many side effects I was experiencing were a direct result of hormonal birth control. I suffered from headaches, mood swing and weight gain. I did not realize the hormones were the cause of my symptoms until I was hormone-free, and my cycles became regular and natural again.

When I was thirty-two, a miscarriage prompted my need for change. I knew I wanted to continue to heal naturally, and I did not want to use hormonal birth control again. In time I was enjoying the regularity of my natural cycles. I felt more energetic and more vibrant than I had in a long time. It felt as though I had been freed of a fog that was clouding my mind. I was thinking more clearly and enjoying life more. However, I still had not figured out the answer to reliable yet natural birth control.

I began my search for natural birth control by talking to doctors and searching on the internet. While searching the internet, I discovered the Yahoo Group DiaphragmsAndCaps, and it was there, where I first learned about female barriers as a reliable form of birth control. It was an online community of like-minded women who were very supportive and helpful on my journey. The advice on the group helped me to seek out what I needed in a doctor, and I went to my first female barrier fitting appointment in October 2003. My first diaphragm was a 65mm Milex Arcing spring. My sizes have varied over the years with weight fluctuation and other factors. I have settled into wearing an 80mm contraceptive diaphragm and an 85 menstrual diaphragm. My cap size varies according to which type of cap. I currently have a wide assortment of caps and diaphragms that I enjoy wearing regularly.

I hope that sharing my story offers guidance and a feeling of comradery to you as you embark on your journey.

CHAPTER 2

∽

CONTRACEPTIVE CHOICES

Contraception is one of the most personal choices a woman will make in her life. The process of choosing a method of contraception is one that requires both time and effort. Birth control is a necessary part of career preparation and family growth management.

There are many choices of contraception available today. The most popular choice among women for many years has been the birth control pill. Vaginal rings, implants, and progestin delivering intra-uterine devices (IUD's) are the other hormonal choices. These methods, though effective, have not been without long and short term side effects and health concerns. Non-hormonal methods include the copper IUD, condoms (male and female), and diaphragms and caps.

No one contraceptive method is perfect, or 100% effective. There are pros and cons to every form of birth control. The best contraceptive choice is one that you and your partner feel comfortable using and one that you will use correctly and consistently. The risk for STI's goes hand in hand with contraceptive decision making. Therefore, it is essential to consider the pros and cons of each method and how they pertain to you as an individual and how you will give yourself STI protection. In general, female barriers have no side effects compared to hormonal or intrauterine methods available on the market.

There are good solid reasons to choose female barriers as your birth control method. The first and foremost is female barriers will give you a safe, effective, all-natural option with no side effects.

Side effects of hormonal birth control include altered menstrual cycles, mood swings, weight gain, depression, headaches, and many more. Most women do not realize they are experiencing side effects from artificial hormones until after they have stopped taking them. While using your diaphragm or cervical cap, you will suffer none of these things as a result of your method. You will always experience the beauty of your natural cycles, and this will make it much easier for you to conceive when you choose to do so.

Throughout your childbearing years (the phase in life that birth control choices seem to be most paramount) your female barriers will protect you from pregnancy as well as from some STI's which can enter your upper reproductive tract and lead to fertility problems. You will also have the added benefit of flow control while using a menstrual diaphragm during menses.

The need to use birth control beyond reproductive years is not something many women consider. Diaphragm and caps should be worn in perimenopause with no change to your regime as the need to protect remains the same(Leitch 1986) (Linton, Golobof et al. 2016). Menopausal women should also continue to wear their caps and dia- phragms for protection from STI's (Carslaw and Cosh 2016). Female barriers allow you to have control over your body in a very natural, safe way throughout your life.

CHAPTER 3

◡

THE INITIAL GYNECOLOGY VISIT

Preparing a young woman for her first gynecology appointment should be given careful consideration. Her initial meeting with a doctor will set the stage for her attitude about follow up care. She should start with the most positive experience possible. Often, if a mother is comfortable and confident in her gynecologist, she will consider taking her daughter to the same practitioner. Having the same physician is potentially ideal and knowing her mother is satisfied with the doctor may help her feel more at ease.

There will always be a certain amount of apprehension attached to a young woman's first gynecological appointment, but there are ways to lessen it. Her mother or a trusted female relative should tell her precisely what to expect at her first appointment. A young lady should know why she is going, what is going to happen once she is there, and have an idea as to what type of birth control she wants to practice before her first appointment. These are practical first steps. Another good idea is to have her meet the doctor beforehand if she does not already know him/her.

The consultation with the health care practitioner is the first step in the fitting appointment. It may be that the mother and daughter will have the initial consultation together if the daughter wishes. Following the discussion, the practitioner will talk to the patient one on one.

The practitioner will stress to the patient that she is in control of the appointment; it is entirely confidential (even from her mother if she wishes). The patient and physician must build a relationship based on trust, which is crucial for the well-being of the patient.

I strongly encourage mothers to talk to their daughters about what to expect and to accompany her to the appointment. It is essential to go over questions and concerns as well as birth control options your daughter is most interested in and to include your wisdom and experience in the conversation. Agree on a doctor or health care practitioner with whom you and your daughter both feel comfortable. If you are satisfied with your male gynecologist, but your daughter wishes to see a female, then it would be in her best interest to seek out a reputable female gynecologist. Nurse practitioners, physician assistants, and naturopaths are often very naturally oriented and supportive of natural birth control options. The more prepared a young woman is for her appointment, and the more involved you are, the better she will feel about it. The better she feels about it initially, the more positive her future experiences will be.

CHAPTER 4

❧

THE FEMALE BARRIER FITTING APPOINTMENT

O nce you have committed to a female barrier method of contraception, it is time to set your focus on the fitting appointment. A correctly fitted barrier is the primary factor in the success of female barrier protection. As there is so much riding on the fit of the diaphragm or cervical cap, you will want to schedule your fitting appointment with the most experienced practitioner you can find.

I recommend calling ahead to inquire about the practitioner's qualifications. The extra effort will ensure you do not spend time and money on an appointment that will not be to your satisfaction. Unfortunately, this may be easier said than done. While this step is useful, you may find yourself continually running into obstacles, which may lead to frustration. I urge you to persevere as the end result will be worth it. In addition to doctors, I suggest nurse practitioners, physician's assistants, and naturopathic doctors as they may be more open to natural methods. Once you have found a qualified practitioner to do your fitting, the hardest part is over!

The following sample questions are a good starting point for researching qualified fitters:

- How many fittings do you do in a week and for how long have you been doing fittings?

- *The practitioner should be doing at least two fittings per week and should have several years of practice.*

- What types of fitting kits do you keep on hand?

- *The practitioner should have diaphragm fitting kits for coil springs and arcing springs and ideally flat springs. He/she should also have cervical cap fitting kits of all types of caps available in your country.*

- Do you fit diaphragms and cervical caps?

- *Ideally, the practitioner should have experience in fitting cervical caps as well as diaphragms. An experienced fitter will provide you with more options in the event your anatomy does not allow you to wear one or the other safely.*

- How long is your initial fitting appointment?

- *A fitting appointment should be at least an hour, ideally one and a half hours to allow time for the diaphragm and or cap fitting as well as the teaching of proper insertion and checking skills.*

- What happens in the fitting appointment?

- *A fitting appointment should cover the pelvic examination, Pap smear and swabs (if indicated) and the diaphragm and or cap fitting itself. Then as long as is needed to teach correct insertion, removal, and protection checks.*

- **Do you schedule a follow up fit check appointment?**

- *Your practitioner should have you schedule an appointment 6-8 weeks after initial fitting and in the fertile window*

- **Do you offer annual fit checks?**

- *The answer should be yes. The practitioner should do an annual fit check. A convenient time for this would be at your yearly well care visit when you get your Pap smear and examination.*

The ideal time to schedule your fitting appointment is during your ovulation window. You need the optimum fit most while you are fertile. In a typical 28 day cycle, this will be on or between cycle day 11 and 16. Ovulation will vary from woman to woman based on her cycle length.

It is not entirely necessary to have the fitting mid-cycle, but it is preferable. Your fitter should do a fit check four weeks after your initial visit to ensure your barrier is the right size and type for you. The follow-up appointment will give you the perfect opportunity to ask any questions you may have since your initial visit. You and your health care practitioner may decide to do an additional menstrual fitting since most women will wear a diaphragm one size larger during their menses for an optimal fit.

Once you have scheduled your fitting appointment, you will want to prepare for the visit. You will be able to get the maximum amount of satisfaction from an informed visit. Many women go to a fitting appointment with certain expectations only to discover it falls short. While it is true the health care staff should be fully prepared to meet your expectations, this is sometimes not the case. The more familiar you are with what should be happening, the more you will be able to contribute to the experience turning out positive. Ask the right questions and leave with the protection that is best for you.

All women should have an updated Pap smear, and barriers users are no exception. The guidelines for cervical cancer screening and birth control prescriptions vary from country to country. In the USA, a woman should have her first Pap smear at age twenty-one. According to the American College Of Gynecologists (Carslaw and Cosh), (2017, 2018), the guidelines for cervical cancer screening are:

- Women aged 21–29 years should have a Pap test alone every three years. HPV testing is not recommended.
- Women aged 30–65 years should have a Pap test and an HPV test (*co-testing*) every five years (preferred). It also is acceptable to have a Pap test alone every three years.

If your Pap smear is not current, your practitioner will do one at the fitting appointment. To be prescribed a cap, you must have a normal Pap smear, but a diaphragm can be worn safely regardless of the result. Once you have been fitted with the correct barriers, the next area of focus will be the type of barrier itself. This decision can seem overwhelming, especially when presented with a lot of information at once. Several factors will help you narrow it down. An excellent place to start would be to examine the choices that are available locally. Ultimately, the best option is the one most suitable for your anatomy as that will provide the safest fit. A great resource is the Yahoo Group DiaphragmsAndCaps, which is where I was very well supported in making my own choice. (Email diaphragmsandcaps-subscribe@yahoogroups.com to subscribe).

If you live in the USA, you will be able to limit your selection to the Cooper Surgical diaphragm or a cervical cap called "FemCap." Your practitioner will let you know which choice is the best fit for you, and you can decide based on that which one or which combination is best for your lifestyle. Many women can safely wear both a FemCap and a diaphragm. You may choose to have both and interchange them throughout your cycle according to what works best for you. I have a variety of different diaphragms and caps that I regularly use at different times in my cycle.

CHAPTER 5

~

FITTING REQUIREMENTS

The proper fit of your cap or diaphragm and user compliance go hand in hand to provide effective female barrier birth control. Your diaphragm or cervical cap should be checked annually for your size and quality of the barrier. Most women have this done at their annual gynecology appointment at the same time they get their Pap smear and breast exam. In addition to a yearly fitting, several things may constitute the need for a fit check.

Weight change is one of the most common reasons for an interim fit check. The diaphragm is more sensitive to weight changes than the cervical cap. Most manufacturers state that a diaphragm should be checked for fit with a weight change of +/- 7 pounds. The rule of thumb is with weight loss a woman will need a larger diaphragm, and with weight gain, she will need a smaller one.

Cervical caps are less sensitive to weight changes. A fit check is required for a weight change of +/- 14 pounds for cavity rim caps such as Prentif and Oves. The FemCap also requires another fitting with a weight change of +/- 14 pounds; however, the situation is a bit more complicated due to the mechanism of how this cap fits. The primary fitting criteria for a FemCap is that the bowl of the cap is large enough to accommodate the cervix adequately. The second fitting criteria is a good seal between the brim of the FemCap and the vaginal wall for the full 360 degrees of the brim. Both requirements must be met for a FemCap to be deemed a safe fit.

When a woman loses weight, the vaginal walls relax, and the vagina becomes larger. The opposite is true when she gains weight. Weight gain would suggest that she would need a smaller cap when she gains weight and a larger cap when she loses weight. The size of the cervix is not affected by weight change to the same degree as the vagina. Weight gain slightly increases the size of the cervix, and weight loss slightly reduces it. When a cap user loses weight, she will most probably (but not always) need a larger size cap. In this case of the FemCap the bowl is also larger and therefore would still fully accommodate the cervix. If she gains weight, she will probably (but not always) need a smaller FemCap for an excellent vaginal wall fit. However, the bowl would also be smaller, and this can often lead to an unsafe fit as the cervix will not fit comfortably into the bowl of the FemCap.

It is also necessary to have the size of your diaphragm or cap checked after giving birth to a baby. The best time to have this done is six-eight weeks postpartum. The degree to which giving birth will affect size varies among women depending on the type of barriers as well as whether the birthing was vaginal or via cesarean section.

If a woman has given birth vaginally and she is a cavity rim cap wearer, it is imperative to have a meticulous examination of the cervix performed to determine if there was any damage sustained to the cervix during the birthing process. If there is any laceration, it may not be possible to continue wearing a cavity rim cap. If this is the case, it may be necessary to switch to a FemCap, Vimule, or Dumas cervical cap or a diaphragm.

In most cases, one of these types of barriers will be a safe option if a cavity rim cap is not. After giving birth vaginally to your first child, your cap or diaphragm size will probably change. A woman commonly stays the same or goes up by one size following the first vaginal birth. If she has given birth via cesarean section, she may stay the same size for her cap or diaphragm, or she may go up. Subsequent births may or may not affect the cap or diaphragm size.

CHAPTER 6

∽

DIAPHRAGMS

The diaphragm is a shallow latex or silicone dome that is placed inside the vagina so that it covers the cervix (the entrance to the uterus) (Roizen, Richardson et al. 2002, 2018). The diaphragm is designed to block semen from entering the cervix. Spermicide (natural or chemical) is placed inside the dome of the diaphragm to immobilize sperm (Roizen, Richardson et al. 2002). The diaphragm must be used together with spermicide and must be left in place six-eight hours post last intercourse to be most effective (Vessey and Wiggins 1974) .

Due to the full range of sizes available, diaphragms are suitable for most women of all ages, body types, and pregnancy history. Diaphragms fit all types of anatomy and are the most commonly prescribed female barrier. They come in a wide range of sizes and rim types and are suitable for women based on their anatomical differences. Most diaphragms used to range in size from 55mm- 95mm, but this range has narrowed over the years due to the lack of popularity of the method. Currently, most diaphragms range in size from 65mm-85mm. Diaphragms have been proven to be more effective than caps for women who have given birth vaginally (Leitch 1986). The cervix can change in size after a vaginal delivery. There is also a possibility that the cervix can suffer damage, and a cap will no longer fit properly. There are more diaphragm types and sizes than there are cap types and sizes, so finding a diaphragm to fit correctly will be much more likely.

Diaphragms are categorized based on rim type and material type. They are manufactured from soft latex rubber or medical grade silicone and are available in arcing, coil, watch spring and flat spring rim types. The best fitting model of diaphragm for you is determined in the fitting appointment and varies from woman to woman based on her anatomy and personal history. The arcing-spring is the most commonly prescribed type of diaphragm as it can be worn safely by women with varying degrees of vaginal muscle tone. Some women can wear multiple rim types safely, specifically those with firm muscle tone.

The **arcing-spring diaphragm** folds into an arc shape when the sides are compressed. The arcing-spring is the strongest and stiffest type of rim available, making it suitable for women with any level of vaginal muscle tone. It has the reputation of being the easiest of all diaphragm types to insert. Examples of the arcing spring diaphragm are:

- **Ortho All-Flex** – Latex and Silicone Diaphragm available in sizes 55-95 mm in steps of 5 mm (no longer in production)

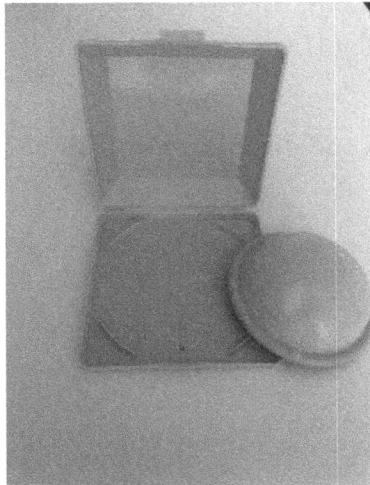

- **Milex Arcing** – Silicone Wide Seal Diaphragm available in sizes 60-90 mm in steps of 5 mm

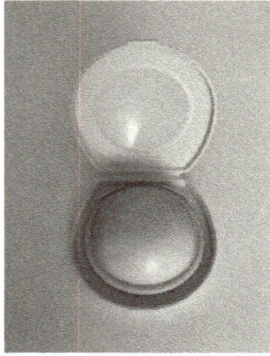

The **coil spring diaphragm** folds into an oval shape and compresses at any point around the rim. This type of rim is not as supportive as that of the arcing- spring type. Because it is not as stiff, it can usually only be worn by women with average to firm vaginal muscle tone. A coil rim type may be a suitable choice for a woman who experiences discomfort with an arcing spring or whose partner experiences discomfort during intercourse.

Examples of coil spring diaphragms are:

- **Semina**– Silicone diaphragm available in sizes 65-85 mm in steps of 5 mm

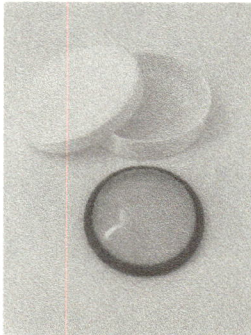

- **Ortho Coil**– Latex diaphragm manufactured in sizes 55-95 mm in steps of 5 mm

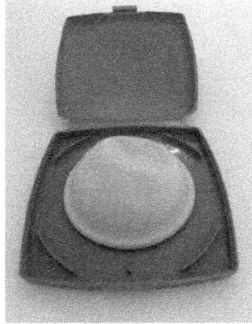

- **Milex Omniflex** – Silicone Wide Seal Diaphragm available in sizes 60-90 mm in steps of 5 mm

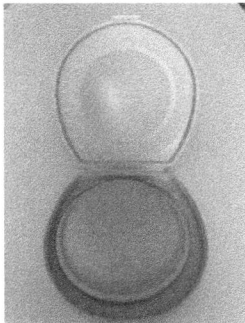

The **flat spring diaphragm** is similar to a coil spring, but the spring is much thinner and only compresses in one plane at any point around the rim. This type of rim is only safe for women with firm vaginal muscle tone.

Examples of flat spring diaphragms are:

- **Reflexions**– Latex diaphragm available in sizes 55-95 mm in 5 mm increments

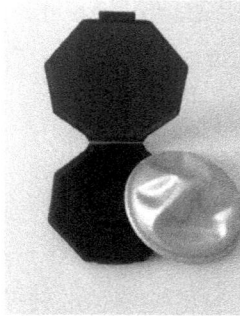

- **Menstrual Diaphragm** - Custom made diaphragms made from natural latex available in a watch or coil spring in sizes 40-110 mm in 2.5 mm steps

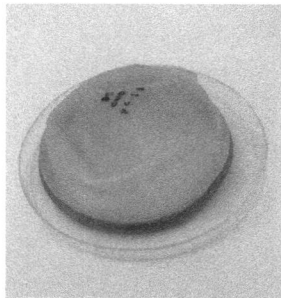

- **Caya Diaphragm (SILCS)** – A new single size contraceptive female barrier that was approved for use in 2013 after an extended trial. It is a contoured diaphragm that is the only one of its type. It is inserted into the vagina the same way a conventional diaphragm or tampon is. Although it is marketed as a one size fits all diaphragm, it is more of one size fits most diaphragm. Unlike a traditional diaphragm, Caya does not have a round shaped rim. The length is 75mm, and the width is 70mm. These dimensions may cause Caya to rotate in women whose conventional diaphragm sizes are above the 70mm – 75mm range.

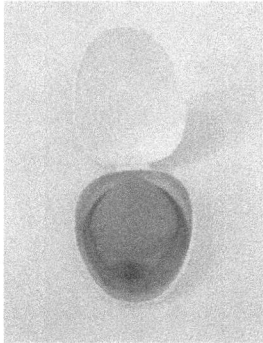

Advantages and Disadvantages of using a Diaphragm

Using a diaphragm has pros and cons, just as any other method of contraception. As a user myself, I have found the advantages far outweigh the disadvantages.

Advantages:

- Statistically more effective than the cervical cap
- Effectiveness is similar to the mini pill or condoms
- No change in the diaphragm's efficiency for women who have given birth vs. women who have not
- Can be inserted several hours before initiation of sexual activity
- Can be used for contraception and flow control during menses
- Approved for a continuous wearing interval of 24 hours before cleaning and reinsertion
- Should not be felt by the user or her partner when correctly fitted and inserted
- Easier to find an experienced fitter
- When used correctly and consistently, the risk of becoming pregnant is less than 2 percent
- Can be inserted several hours before initiation of sexual activity

- Hormone-free
- Offer protection against some STI's
- Less expensive than many other methods of birth control
- Can be reused and may last for several years depending on the frequency of use and proper car

Disadvantages:

- Must be fitted for a diaphragm by a healthcare professional
- Must use spermicide (chemical or natural)
- Insertion may interrupt sex
- Must always be available during travel
- Practice is needed to learn to insert a diaphragm correctly and quickly
- An incorrectly fitted diaphragm, specifically a diaphragm that is too large, may contribute to bladder or urinary tract infections if the wearer is prone to them

Contraindications:

- If the muscles in your vagina are not firm enough to hold the diaphragm in place
- If you have an unusual shape or position of the cervix, the practitioner will advise about this when they examine you for correct fitting
- If you are very overweight, fitting may be difficult in this case.
- If you have given birth within the previous six weeks, this is because your body has not had a chance to get back to normal. The fit may change once you are back to normal.
- If you are allergic or sensitive to rubber (latex) or spermicide.
- If you have ever had toxic shock syndrome, you should be cautious

- If you have HIV or AIDS (or are at high risk of HIV infection) The reason for this is because diaphragms and caps should be used with spermicides, and people with HIV or AIDS should not use spermicides.

Instructions for Diaphragm Insertion:
- For maximum efficacy, you must always use a diaphragm in conjunction with spermicide. Some women may choose to insert a diaphragm every night to avoid the chance of having unprotected intercourse and risk an unplanned pregnancy.

- Inspect the diaphragm for holes by holding it up to a light. If there are holes or defects, the diaphragm will not work effectively, even with a spermicide. It must be replaced.

- Before you put the diaphragm over the cervix (opening to the uterus), a spermicide cream, foam, gel, or jelly should be put into the cup of the diaphragm. Follow the manufacturer's directions on how much spermicide to use and how long before sexual intercourse you may apply the spermicide.

- Also, spread some spermicide all around the rim of the diaphragm that will be touching the cervix. Some health care practitioners advise spreading more spermicide on the outside of the cup of the diaphragm.

- To insert the diaphragm, squeeze the rim between your thumb and forefinger so that it is narrow enough to fit into the vagina. Be careful if you have long nails as you may nick the latex or silicone of the diaphragm or you may scratch yourself. Wearing gloves with long nails will help to avoid that problem. While in a comfortable position, push the diaphragm as deeply into the vagina as it will go and release the rim. Some women use an applicator that makes it easier to insert the diaphragm. The diaphragm rim should be round again and back of the rim directly behind the cervix. The front of the rim should be pushed up behind the public bone.

- For each additional act of intercourse, you must add an extra applicator full of spermicide into the vagina (5 ml).
- Do not remove the diaphragm if it has been in place less than 6 or 8 hours since the last sexual intercourse. For the diaphragm to be most effective at preventing pregnancy. Be careful not to move the diaphragm out of place while you are applying more spermicide.
- Wearing a diaphragm for more than 24 hours increases the risk of toxic shock syndrome or a urinary tract infection.
- To remove the diaphragm, hook one finger over the front of the rim. Pull the diaphragm downward and out of the vagina.

CHAPTER 7

∼

CERVICAL CAPS

The cervical cap is a dome-shaped device that fits snugly over the cervix. The cap is a barrier which blocks the passage of sperm from the vagina through the cervix into the uterus and tubes where they can fertilize the ripened egg. Cervical caps are used with a small amount of natural or chemical spermicide. The natural spermicides are lactic acid-based, aloe and lemon juice or honey. Cervical caps must be left in place for at least 6 hours post last intercourse. A Pap smear is required within 6 months before fitting a cervical cap to ensure the cervix is healthy and not damaged. Cervical caps are smaller than diaphragms and they do not interfere with the bladder. They can be left in place for more extended periods compared to diaphragms (Parenthood 2016).

Cervical caps are excellent choices for a lot of women. They are the less common choice, mostly because of availability and because of practioners' lack of knowledge in fitting them. When the Prentif was availabe in the USA, caps were more often prescribed over diaphragms. The Prentif was taken off,the market in the USA because the cost to renew the medical device license,was prohibitive even with a high demand for the cap. The demand remains to this day, and some women travel abroad for Prentif cap fittings. Today in the USA the only cap currently available is the FemCap.

A cervical cap differs from a diaphragm in that it is much smaller and can be worn for more extended periods (up to 72 hours) between cleaning and reinsertion and does not need additional spermicide applications with each act of intercourse. For many women, the length of time a barrier can be worn is a factor in determining personal wearing regime. It can be the difference as to whether you prefer a cap over a diaphragm.

The two main types of cervical caps are cavity rim and vaginal vault. Cervical caps are made from natural latex or medical grade silicone the same as diaphragms. There are three latex reusable types (Prentif, Vimule, and Dumas), one reusable silicone type (Femcap) and one silicone single-use disposable type (Oves). Although Oves was marketed as a disposable cap, many users have had success reusing the Oves since its removal from the market in 2010 (2011). The cavity rim cap, such as Prentif or Oves, has a cavity on the inside of the rim which creates a seal and keeps the cap in place together with the support of the vaginal wall. A raised rim protrusion on the cervix when the cap is removed indicates a perfect fit. The vaginal vault cap, such as Vimule, FemCap, and Dumas, forms a seal by adhering to the vaginal wall.

- **FemCap:** Silicone cap available in 22mm, 26mm, 30mm

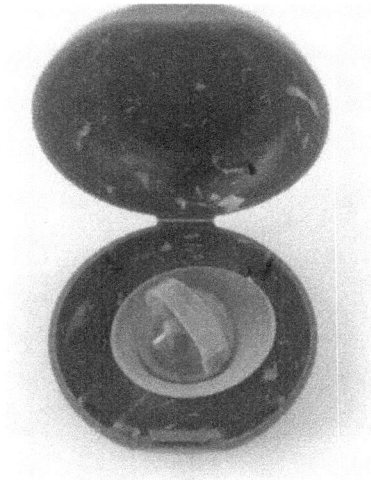

- **Vimule:** Latex vault cap manufactured in sizes 42, 48, and 52 mm

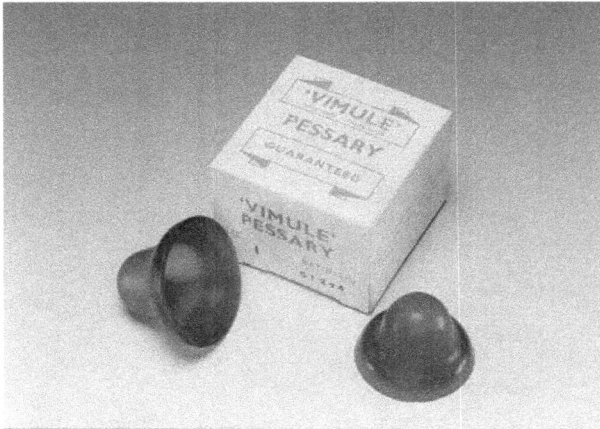

- **Dumas:** Latex cap manufactured in five sizes: 50, 55, 60, 65, and 75mm external diameter

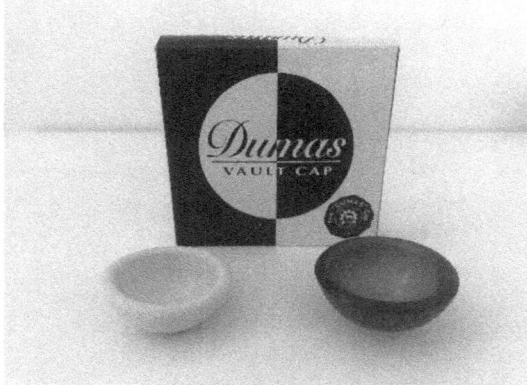

- **Oves:** Silicone cavity rim cap available in 22mm, 26mm, 30mm
The Oves is a unique fitting cavity rim cap. It adheres to the cervix in the same fashion as the Prentif and forms a cavity rim raised ring around the cervix. The raised ring is an indication of a good fit. The Oves is unique in that the silicone dome adheres to the cervix much like saran wrap on a bowl.

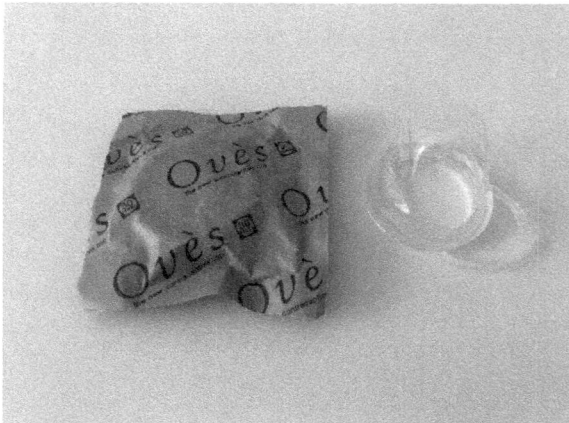

- **Prentif:** Latex cavity rim cap available in 22mm, 25mm, 28mm, 31mm

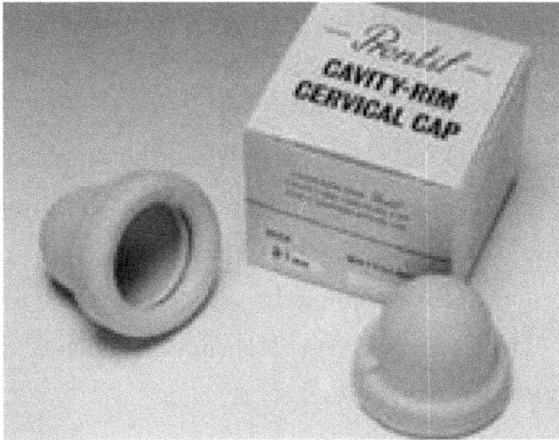

- **Metal Caps**: metal caps available in 2 mm increments ranging in size from 20mm to 30mm
  This type of cap has recently become available in hard plastic. Currently, only available in China.

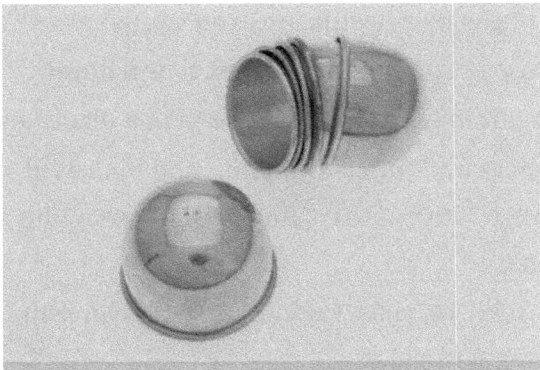

Advantages and Disadvantages of using a Cervical Cap
Advantages:
- Can remain inserted for up to 3 days (5 days if used with honey) allowing spontaneous protected sex
- Continuous regimes are available
- Smaller and use less spermicide than the diaphragm
- Protect against pregnancy for multiple acts of intercourse without additional applications of spermicide
- Often can be worn when a diaphragm does not fit well
- When placed correctly, cervical caps are often not felt by either partner
- No hormonal side effects
- Can be used with natural spermicides
- Protects against certain STI's
- Does not contribute to urinary tract or bladder infections

Disadvantages:
- Requires fitting by a healthcare professional
- Requires use of spermicide (chemical or natural)
- More difficult to insert and remove than a diaphragm
- Odor, unpleasant vaginal discharge, and increased TSS risk can occur if worn for over three days without cleaning

Contraindications:
- If the muscles in your vagina are not firm enough to hold the diaphragm in place
- If you have an unusual shape or position of the cervix, the practitioner will advise about this when they examine you for correct fitting

- If your BMI is high, fitting may be difficult in this case
- If you have given birth within the previous six weeks, this is because your body has not had a chance to get back to normal The fit may change once you are back to normal
- If you have ever had TSS
- If you have cancer of the cervix, or are being treated for abnormal Pap smears
- If you have HIV or AIDS (or are at high risk of HIV infection) The reason is that diaphragms and caps should be used with spermicides, and spermicides should not be used by those with HIV or AIDS. (1982)

Instructions for Cervical Cap Insertion:

- For maximum efficacy, cervical caps must always be used with a spermicide. Some women may choose to insert a diaphragm every night to avoid the chance of having unprotected intercourse and risk an unplanned pregnancy.
- Inspect the cap for holes by holding it up to a light. If there are holes or defects, the diaphragm will not work effectively, even with a spermicide. It must be replaced.
- Before you put the cap over the cervix (opening to the uterus), a spermicide cream, foam, gel, or jelly should be put into the dome of the cap. Follow the manufacturer's directions on how much spermicide to use (usually dome 1/3 full) and how long before sexual intercourse you should insert your cap (usually 15 mins). Also, when using the FemCap health care practitioners advise spreading more spermicide on the outside of the bowl.
- To insert the cap squeeze between your thumb and forefinger so that it is narrow enough to fit into the vagina. Be careful if you have long nails as you may nick the latex or silicone of the

cap or you may scratch yourself. Wearing gloves with long nails will help to avoid that problem. While in a comfort- able position, push the cap in as deeply into the vagina as it will go and check to see if it has covered the cervix. Cavity rim caps should be given a ¼ turn on the cervix to maximise the cavity rim seal.

- For every additonal act of intercourse, you must add an extra applicator full of spermicide into the vagina (5 ml) if you are using the FemCap or Dumas cap. Additional spermicide is not necessary if you are wearing a cavity rim cap.

- Do not remove the cervical cap if it has been less than 6 or 8 hours since the last sexual intercourse. For the cap to be most effective at preventing pregnancy, it must remain in the vagina for at least 6 or 8 hours post intercourse. Be careful not to move the Femcap or Dumas out of place while you are adding more spermicide.

- To remove the cap, hook one finger over the rim or pull at the dome to release the suction. Pull the cap downward and out of the vagina.

CHAPTER 8

∽

INTERNAL CONDOMS

The internal condom is a barrier method of contraception that is used to prevent pregnancy and STI's. It is a lubricated sheath similar in shape to that of a male condom, but it is wider. It is available in both latex and polyurethane. The internal condom is very convenient as an over the counter product, and unlike a cap or diaphragm does not require a prescription or fitting. Any woman can wear any type and size despite changes in weight or with pregnancy history. It allows the woman to have complete control over the method with very few side effects.

When worn during intercourse, the internal condom lines the entire interior of the vagina and covers the labia, thereby preventing semen from entering the uterus and fertilizing an egg. By shielding the walls of the vagina and labia from semen and other bodily fluids, the internal condom is very effective at preventing STI's (Roizen, Richardson et al. 2002).

The internal condom is inserted into the vagina with the open end left on the outside.. The device at the closed end of the sheath is used to insert the condom into the vagina and to hold it in place during intercourse. In some types, the closed end against the cervix has a flexible ring similar to the rim of a small diaphragm. In other models, the closed end has a sponge or dissolvable insert. The rolled outer ring at the open end of the sheath remains outside the vagina and covers the external genitalia. Internal condoms on the market today do not contain any spermicide. The latex versions give better heat transfer than the polyurethane versions.

Many couples prefer the feeling of latex because it is a more natural, skin to skin feeling and provides better heat transfer. There are advantages and disadvantages to every method. Below is a list you can use to assist you in deciding if the internal condom is right for you.

There are several different types and sizes of internal condoms available today, including panty versions. For most women, a medium sized condom is adequate. However, women who have recently given birth should try a large size first. Any size will work for any woman, but it is a matter of specific sizes being more comfortable than others.

The original version of internal condom (brand names included Reality, Femy, and Femidom), was made of polyurethane. Large-scale production of the nitrile FC2 began in 2007. The FDA approved the condom in March 2009. Now there are several versions of polyurethane internal condoms as well as latex versions (Wing 2016)

Below is a detailed list of the internal condoms currently available:

Polyurethane:

- **FC2**: nitrile sheath 17 cm (6.7 in) in length. There is a flexible ring at either end. At the closed end of the sheath, the pliable ring is inserted into the vagina to hold the internal condom in place. The other end of the sheath stays outside the vulva at the entrance to the vagina. This ring acts as a guide during penetration and stops the sheath from shifting during intercourse. There is a silicone-based lubricant on the inside of the condom, but additional lubrication can be used. The condom does not contain spermicide

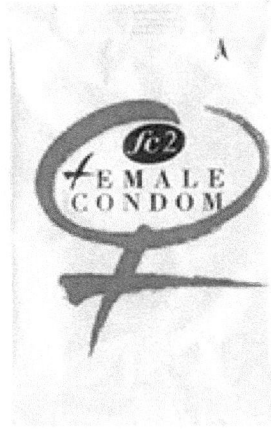

- **The Woman's Condom:** developed by PATH, through a user-centered design process is a relatively new internal condom. The Woman's Condom is a polyurethane pouch that is partially enclosed in a capsule to aid insertion. The tablet dissolves quickly after insertion in the vagina, which releases the pouch. The condom is then held stable in the woman by foam pads. The Woman's Condom is packaged dry and comes with a small sachet of water-based lubricant to be applied at the point of use. WHO is currently reviewing the Woman's Condom.

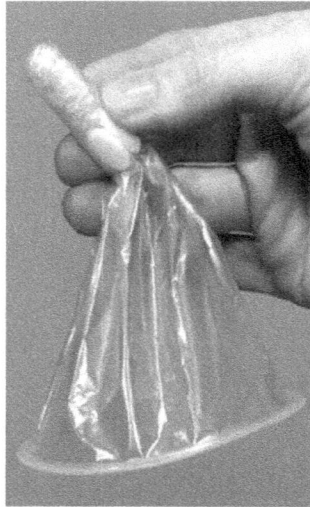

- **The Natural Sensation Panty Condom:** distributed in the US exclusively by the ACME Condom Company. Natural Sensation Compañia Ltda manufactures it. (NS) Based in Bogotá, Colombia. The product is made of a polyethylene resin, which is stronger and thinner than latex. Unlike latex, polyethylene is hypo-allergenic, transparent, and odorless. Natural Sensation's condoms are lubricated and may be used with either oil- or water-based lubricants.

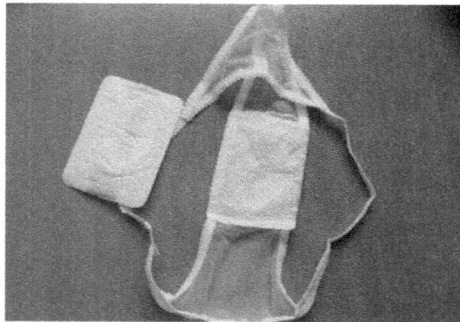

- **The Phoenurse:** made of a dumb-bell shaped polyurethane sheath and comes with an insertion tool, water- based or silicone-based lubricant, sanitary towels, and disposal bags. The Tianjin Condombao Medical Polyurethane Tech. Co. Ltd.is the manufacturer and the condom is approved for sale in Europe. It is available in Brazil, Sri Lanka, China, Kenya, and Mexico. The FDA has not yet approved it.

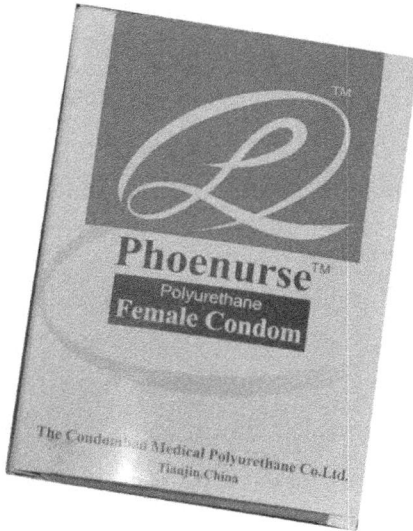

Latex:

- **The VA w.o.w.:** (worn-of-women) condom has a latex pouch attached to its rounded triangular outer frame, with soft sponge inside the pouch that secures it firmly inside the vagina. Its one size fits all design fits the outer shell snugly against the external female genitalia, providing a protective latex shield to prevent skin-to-skin contact between partners. It is available worldwide, and currently online at several locations, including eBay for direct home delivery anywhere in the world, with free shipping. The VA w.o.w internal condom is CE Mark-approved through its Indian manufacturer, HLL Ltd., a govt of India enterprise.

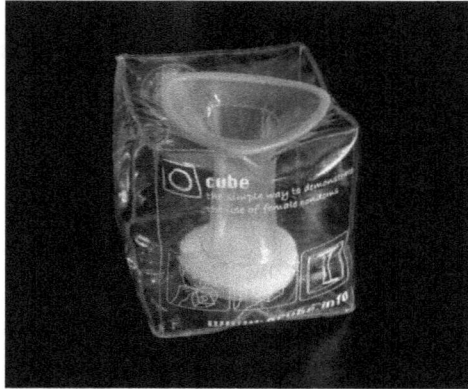

- **The Female Panty Condom:** Latex condom manufactured by Silk Parasol. Not yet FDA approved and is currently undergoing clinical trials. The Panty Condom is a panty with a replaceable pantyliner containing a condom made of synthetic resin. The man's penis inserts the condom, and the panty itself can be reused with another condom for additional acts of intercourse.

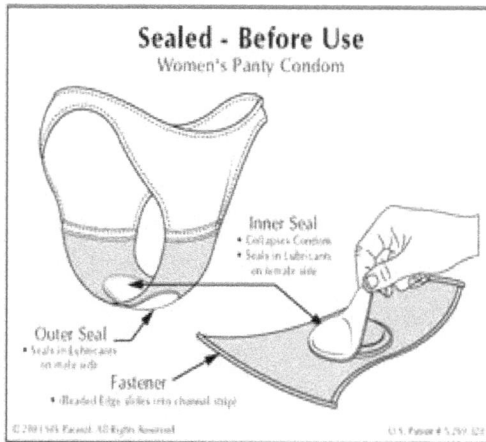

- **The Cupid Angel Internal Condom:** Made of latex and manufactured in India by Cupid Ltd. It is approved for distribution in Europe and was prequalified for distribution by WHO in 2012. It is currently undergoing clinical trials to gain approval from the FDA.

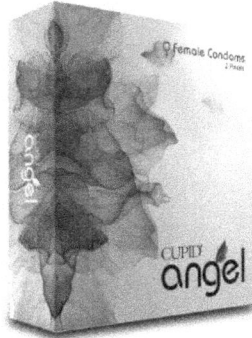

Advantages and Disadvantages of using an Internal Condom

There are advantages and disadvantages to every method. Below is a list you can use to assist you in deciding if the internal condom is right for you.

Advantages:

- Can be inserted at any time ahead of intercourse
- Very high level of protection against STI's such as gonorrhea, syphilis, chlamydia, HIV, and HPV
- Entirely under the female's control
- Hormone free
- The receptive partner can use internal condoms during anal sex
- Requires no fitting or prescription
- Can be used with a cervical cap for dual protection

Disadvantages:

- May cause irritation of the genital area in either the male or female partner
- May reduce sensation during intercourse
- Squeaky noise with the polyurethane types

Internal condoms are a very convenient and safe method of birth control for women. It is a very effective option and readily available to women in all parts of the world. It is very convenient for women to purchase them as they are sold over the counter at most pharmacies, just as male condoms are. Internal condoms allow a safer range of use than caps or diaphragms, but a woman can experiment to find what is best for her. Internal condoms are a very effective method of birth control and STI protection, and they have a way of providing women with a sense of control over contraception.

CHAPTER 9

~

SPERMICIDES

Vaginal spermicide is a type of contraception that immobilizes sperm before it reaches the egg. Its purpose is to prevent fertilization. It is one of the oldest forms of contraception on record dating back to Egyptian times. Back then, the type of spermicide used was made of crocodile dung and fermented dough . Today spermicide is much more evolved. It is now available in the forms of creams, jellies, foams, films, suppositories, and sponges. Spermicide can be used alone, but it is considerably less effective than using it as part of a combined method. Combined methods, such as a diaphragm and or a cap and spermicide, result in lower rates of pregnancy than using either method by itself (Farr, Gabelnick et al. 1994).

Spermicide is an essential part of female barrier use. It is necessary to use spermicide together with your cap or diaphragm for the barrier to be most effective. Clinical studies involving caps and diaphragms all included the use of spermicide . Sometimes it may seem like a hassle or an extra step, but it is a necessary one. This is particularly true for younger couples and those with a high level of fertility(Farr, Gabelnick et al. 1994)(Farr, Gabelnick et al. 1994)(Farr, Gabelnick et al. 1994)(Farr, Gabelnick et al. 1994). Spermicide comes in many different forms: creams, gels, film, foams, and suppositories (soft inserts that melt into cream inside the vagina). Spermicide can be broken down into two main categories: 1.) Chemical and 2.) Natural.

Chemical spermicides are sold over the counter and are available in most pharmacies and chain stores. They are very easy to obtain as they do not require a prescription. The active ingredient in most spermicides is nonoxynol-9 (N-9). Other chemical components used for spermicides include Benzalkonium Chloride, Chlorhexidine, Menfegol, Octoxynol-9, and Sodium Docusate.

Natural ingredient spermicides can be purchased through various online sites and can be made at home. The main components are lactic acid, lemon juice, and honey. Many women experience sensitivity to N-9 or other inactive ingredients found in spermicide or develop infections after use. The reason this happens is the active ingredient, N-9, can alter the pH balance of the vagina by destroying favorable bacteria, which keeps the vaginal flora in balance. Natural spermicides do not have this effect.

On the contrary, they help to maintain the proper pH balance in the vagina and aid in preventing infections. Women who use chemical spermicides with their caps, diaphragms, and condoms should make a routine of douching regularly to maintain normal vaginal pH levels. Douching is less critical for natural spermicide users as the pH of the vagina remains unaltered. Spermicide of any type does not protect against STI's.

Chemical Spermicides:
- Advantage-S
- Conceptrol
- Delfen Foam
- Emko
- Encare
- First-Progressive VGS

- Gynol II - Jelly
- Today Sponge
- VCF-Vaginal Contraceptive Film

Natural Spermicides:

- Aloe Vera Lemon Juice
- Lemon Juice, Honey & Corn Starch
- Manuka Honey - must be minimum UMF 16 +
- Contragel - 2 percent lactic acid
- Femprotect – 3 percent lactic acid

Advantages and Disadvantages of using Spermicide

ADVANTAGES:

- Effective in preventing pregnancy when used in conjunction with another barrier method
- No lasting effect on a woman's natural hormones
- No prescription is required
- Inexpensive and readily available

DISADVANTAGES:

- Less effective when used as the only method
- No clear evidence of STI protection
- Requires interruption of sexual activity
- Some may consider it messy
- Must be reapplied for every additional act of intercourse
- Some people experience irritation or allergic reactions

Spermicides should be stored in a cool, dry place, if possible, out of the sun. Suppositories may melt in hot weather. If kept dry, foaming tablets are not as likely to melt in hot weather.

CHAPTER 10

$\sim$

MENSTRUAL PROTECTION

U sing a menstrual diaphragm can be a liberating experience. It may sound unusual at first, especially to those of us who are used to conventional pads and tampons. Pads are useful at times, but a diaphragm for flow control is very functional and convenient. A menstrual diaphragm offers its users a wide variety of flexibility and excellent protection for flow control and contraception. Not unlike a diaphragm that is used in the traditional sense, a menstrual diaphragm requires a proper fitting appointment by your health care practitioner. A menstrual diaphragm with the correct fit will provide maximum protection for flow control as well as for contraception.

Among the benefits of a menstrual diaphragm is the user's ability to have intercourse during her menses. Of course, a woman can continue to have sex during her period even if she is not a barrier user, but it is safer and less messy when a diaphragm is used. There are also several types of menstrual cups on the market today, but none are designed for or approved as safe for use during intercourse. That may be the primary reason female barrier users embrace their menstrual diaphragms.

The diaphragm is very useful for flow control provided it is the right size and rim type. You can exercise, swim, and do any activity you can do while wearing a pad or tampon, without the exposure to harmful chemicals which are often present in tampons or pads.

Most women find a diaphragm more comfortable than wearing bulky pads. Menstrual diaphragm use is also safer for the environment as it reduces the amount of waste sent back to the earth. The diaphragm is reusable for many years, which makes it more cost-effective as well.

Menstrual diaphragms can be either latex or silicone, the same as a contraceptive diaphragm. Most women will wear a diaphragm that is one size larger than the diaphragm they use during their fertile window, so it is a good idea to have a menstrual fitting in addition to an ovulatory fitting. Increase in size during menses is simply a guideline and will not be accurate in every case. The diaphragm will eventually stain as the result of continued exposure to blood, especially if it is latex, but this will in no way hinder the effectiveness.

Diaphragms for menstrual flow control are convenient and safe. Many women have two diaphragms, one for birth control and one for contraception and flow control during menses. A diaphragm can be used alone or in conjunction with a pad or panty liner for extra protection from leakage. I often hear women prefer to avoid intercourse during their menses, or even more frequently that their partners prefer to abstain. A diaphragm for flow control decreases the mess or leakage many couples are deterred by, and a well fitted menstrual diaphragm will eliminate leakage provided it is emptied before it becomes full. Many patients who have switched from tampons or pads to a menstrual diaphragm are much happier and experience more freedom in the day to day activities. A menstrual diaphragm can be worn during any regular activity, including exercise and swimming.

A diaphragm should be reinserted and cleaned at least every twenty-four hours, and this is especially important during menses. Old blood can contribute to an increased risk for TSS because menstrual blood allows vaginal bacteria to multiply unless the diaphragm is cleaned at least every 24 hours. This problem is usually not linked with menstrual diaphragm use as it is emptied several times a day or at least once a day on light flow days.

Latex or silicone diaphragms may be used during menses, but silicone, which is increasing in popularity among all users, is an excellent choice because it does not stain as easily as latex and it is less likely to develop odors. Depending on the size of the diaphragm, most women find they need to empty their diaphragm every 4-6 hours. Draining time varies widely and depends on cycle day, how heavy the flow is, as well as the diaphragm size. Larger diaphragms hold significantly more menstrual flow than smaller ones. On lighter days the diaphragm can be emptied less often.

CHAPTER 11

~

PERSONAL WEARING REGIMES

O nce your fitting is over, the most challenging part is upon you. You have made your decision, you have had your fitting, and you are motivated! You have your diaphragm or cervical cap in your possession (perhaps both), and you are ready to experiment. You are feeling excited yet nervous about using your new barriers. There is always a learning curve, but once you master the skill, you will feel confident and in control.

As a new user, it is only natural that you will feel apprehensive and inadequately protected during the learning phase. This is a prevalent feeling among new barrier users. The more you practice, the more assured you will feel that you are using your barriers correctly and that they provide you with reliable, safe protection. Some women who can safely wear both a cavity rim cap, such as Oves or Prentif, and a diaphragm choose to wear them both at the same time. This is especially common with new users and with women who want added protection during their ovulation window.

It is necessary to select a wearing regime that conforms to your lifestyle. If you do not wear your barrier correctly and consistently, it is not going to prevent pregnancy. There are perfect use statistics and typical use statistics (see appendix C). You want to be as close to a perfect user as you possibly can. In partnership with your healthcare provider, you should strive to develop a wearing regime that will comfortably fit into your lifestyle and become a routine part of your daily life.

Whether you have one barrier or multiple barriers, it is essential to keep them in a convenient location readily available to you when you are likely to need them. For most women, this place is the bathroom or the bedroom. Women who prefer a continuous regime often like to clean and reinsert during their showers. Women who prefer to use their barriers on an as-needed basis may favor their caps and diaphragms to be stored in the bedroom nightstand. Another popular choice is a purse and travel bag. The critical element is always to have your cap or diaphragm available when you need it!

There are two schools of thought as far as barrier wearing is concerned. One focuses on using barriers on an as-needed basis, and the other focuses on continuous wearing routines. Another popular routine is the "weekend" wearing regime where barriers are worn continuously from Friday to Monday and on an as-needed basis from Tuesday until Friday.

Ladies may prefer to wear their barriers on an as-needed basis because it fits well into their lifestyles. It can be that a woman does not live with her partner or that one or the other travels; therefore, does not expect to have intercourse daily. For women who choose this wearing regime, carrying in the purse or travel bag is paramount for safety and successful barrier protection.

Purses come in all shapes and sizes as do the women who carry them. A woman's purse is her sacred domain. It can be private, cluttered, and even mysterious in its contents. In it, she carries her makeup, her wallet, her credit cards, her hairbrush, her lotion and pictures of her loved ones. Inside she will find a tissue, gum, candy, panty liners, sanitary pads, and the list goes on and on.

I have a purse suitable for every season and occasion in all shapes and sizes! I may even have as many purses as I do caps and diaphragms. Purses and travel bags also play an essential role for women whose lifestyles are better suited to continuous barrier wearing regime.

Women who carry diaphragms and cervical caps often carry a supply of condoms as well. Diaphragm and cervical cap cases are compact and discreet and can fit well and unnoticeably in just about any purse or travel bag. The diaphragm case is similar in size and shape to a makeup compact. Discretion is desired by most, but on occasion, there is the user who likes to display the fact that she wears a diaphragm or cervical cap.

I am an organized person with an ordinary daily routine. I have applicators, spermicides, and condoms all arranged in a specific order. I like to reinsert, clean, and switch my female barrier daily. I enjoy the variety of picking out and changing to a suitable cap or diaphragm for my cycle day. If I am menstrual, or shortly will menstruate, I will pick one of my diaphragms suitable for menstrual use. If I am ovulatory, I will select one of my caps.

I am a continuous barrier wearer, but I still like to have an extra diaphragm or cap in my purse. I always feel more confident taking a spare item for when I have unexpected bleeding, or I need to change the one I am wearing. Make sure to take the time you need to develop your own wearing regime, and do not be discouraged if takes a while to figure out. Before you know it, you will be an expert user confident in your method!.

CHAPTER 12

∾

DOUCHING

It is a good practice for female barrier users to douche, especially for those who have had problems with vaginal infections. For anyone who uses chemical spermicides, this is especially important because the N-9 "kills" the good bacteria in the vagina as well as the sperm; therefore, increasing the chance of infections among barrier users. Douching will help the vagina to remain healthy by keeping the vaginal pH in normal balance. Douching is a good practice for vaginal hygiene, whether you are a barrier user or not as long as you stick to a formula that is the exact normal pH of the vagina. The problem arises when using premixed solutions that are not pH balanced such as some of the ones found in stores. Anything that is perfumed and has any ingredient other than water and vinegar is not recommended.

The most convenient way to douche is to purchase a 'travel douche bag.' A travel douche bag is a small (12oz usually) folding latex bag with a removable nozzle and a carrying case such as the one depicted here which is available on Amazon.

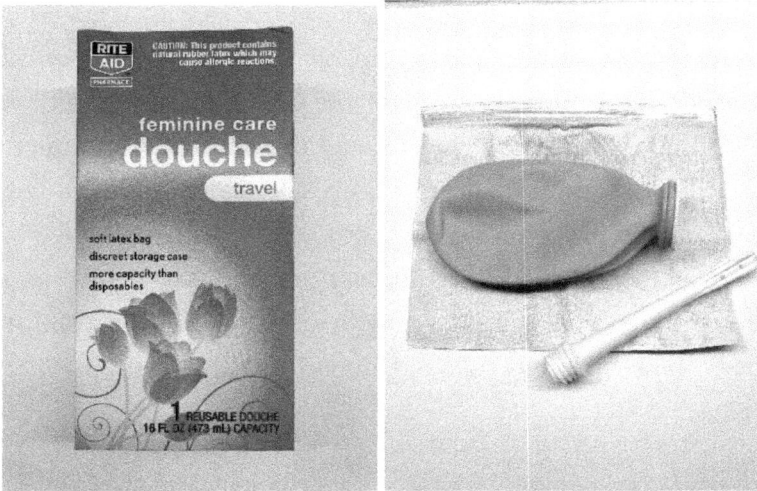

When preparing your douching mixture, you will want to use a 10:1 distilled water to white vinegar solution, which is the exact pH as a healthy vagina and will not cause any infection or irritation. The white vinegar should be the distilled type and ideally organic (should contain no petroleum products). It's best to put 1 part (1 oz) white vinegar into the douche bag directly and then fill the rest of the bag with warm water. I keep a small bottle of vinegar in my bathroom, so it is conveniently on hand.

You should not douche until it is time to remove your cap or diaphragm, which is a minimum of 6 hours post last intercourse. Use one half the douche mixture before removing your cap or diaphragm (this will help wash out any bacteria introduced by the male partner) and the other half after it has been removed. If you are not a regular barrier user, it is recommended to douche once in a cycle on the day after menstrual bleeding stops and then only as needed and not routinely.

Douching is helpful if you have had problems with yeast infections and balancing vaginal pH. For anyone who uses chemical spermicides, this is especially important because the N9 "kills" the good bacteria in the vagina as well as the sperm and therefore has the potential to increase infections among barrier users. Douching will help keep the vagina healthy while using barriers, and it is a good practice for vaginal hygiene, whether you are a barrier user or not. If you feel comfortable with douching (some women are while others are not) it is important to douche the proper way to avoid any infection or irritation by maintaining proper vaginal pH.

CHAPTER 13

~

CLEANING & STORAGE OF BARRIERS

Diaphragms and cervical caps, both latex and silicone, require proper care to ensure the best protection for you and longer life for the barrier. A diaphragm or cervical cap may last for many years, depending on the frequency of use and storage conditions. Typically, silicone has a longer wearing life than latex, but this varies widely depending on the amount of use the barrier gets. Silicone is impervious to petroleum and oil-based creams and lubricants. It is recommended to have female barriers examined professionally at least once a year. The perfect opportunity for this would be at your annual exam when you have your fitting check. It is also good practice to check your barriers on your own at home.

Most female barrier users have more than one diaphragm or cervical cap for various reasons. At the very least a woman needs one diaphragm or cervical cap for contraception, and another diaphragm to wear for menstrual contraception and flow control. This is the most practical and safest option. Some women prefer a wider variety of cervical barriers for convenience or personal preference. Many women like to keep cervical barriers stored in their purses or travel bags, reducing the likelihood of not being prepared when necessary.

It is common for your menstrual diaphragm to become stained over time, and occasionally you may notice the diaphragm develops an odor. Staining is far more noticeable and happens more quickly with latex barriers than with silicone.

With time and use, both latex, as well as silicone, will eventually become stained. The stain in no way affects the durability of the diaphragm. However, you must frequently check your barrier for holes or weak spots indicated by hardening, dimpling, or rippling in the latex or silicone. Inspect the diaphragm or cap for holes by holding it up to a light or by running water through it and inspecting it for drips. If you notice any of these, it will be necessary to replace the barrier right away as it could easily fail during use even with the use of spermicide.

It is essential to follow the manufacturers' cleaning and storage instructions that accompany your cervical barrier. For everyday cleaning of your caps and diaphragms, regular soap and warm water is recommended. Always try to avoid scented soaps. Never use talcum powder on your latex barriers as this will contribute to the deterioration of the latex. It is preferable to store your barriers in their original cases when not in use, and always be sure to allow your cap or diaphragm to dry completely before closing the storage case. Your supplies should be stored in an area that is clean, cool, dark, and, most importantly, convenient for you.

There are times when you will notice your barrier may have an odor, and you will have to disinfect it. Several options are effective and will not cause damage to the caps or diaphragms. Vinegar is a common disinfecting agent. Women find it preferable because it is a household item and usually readily on hand. Latex and silicone barriers may be soaked in vinegar for 10 minutes or 50/50 vinegar/water for 30 minutes to sterilize and remove the odor. Another option would be to use bleach.

A 1:3 bleach and water mixture for 10 minutes is effective and will eliminate odor, but when bleach is used, the barriers can be left in the solution no longer than thirty minutes. Milton's is the preferred sterilizing solution that can be bought in stores or online https://www.milton-tm.com/en/consumer/products/sterilising-fluid. It is marketed as a baby bottle sterilizing solution, so it is gentle and effective and can be safely used for all types of diaphragms and caps. Any product that is comparable to Milton's may be used as a substitution. Caring for the barriers will pay off in longevity and safety.

CHAPTER 14

~

PROTECTION FOR THE FEMALE COUPLE

Female barriers play a significant role when it comes to the topic of safe sex for females couples and bisexual women . Protection for female couples and bisexual women is in every way as relevant as it is to heterosexual couples. Female barrier protection not only protects from pregnancy but also some STI's .

Bisexual women have the same protection needs as heterosexual women. They require protection from pregnancy as well as STI's. They need to use a female barrier to protect from pregnancy as well as a male or internal condom for full STI protection. While pregnancy may not be a concern for same-sex couples, the issue for STI protection is. Safe sex via female barriers is a way to protect from contracting or transmitting STI's, including but not limited to HPV and HIV.

To ensure each partner is equally protected each member of the female couple should practice the use of female barriers for every act of intercourse. Female barriers include a diaphragm or cervical cap to protect the cervix from HPV and to protect the tubes from harmful diseases, such as Chlamydia and Gonorrhea. To fully protect from all STI's, it is necessary for the female couple to incorporate an internal condom.

For dildos, vibrators and other sex toys, it is required to add a male condom, particularly if the items are shared.

CHAPTER 15

∾

SEXUAL HEALTH

S exual health is an essential consideration when making birth control choices. Most methods today focus primarily on the prevention of pregnancy. A sexually active woman must equally consider protection against STI's as well as pregnancy. Sometimes the former is overlooked as the consequences of an unplanned pregnancy seem more immediate than those of contracting an STI. The result of an STI can be just as devastating or more so because if left untreated can result in health issues ranging from cervical cancer to infertility. The most prominent STI's are HPV, Chlamydia, and Gonorrhea .

HPV is a sexually transmitted virus that has the potential to cause serious cervical disease. It affects both males and females. Fourteen strains of high-risk HPV are contracted sexually. High-risk strains of HPV (primarily 6,11,16, 18, 31,33,45, 52 and 58 which account for over 90 percent of cervical cancer cases) (Lehfeldt, Sobrero et al. , Quarini 2005) (Lehfeldt, Sobrero et al. , Quarini 2005) (Lehfeldt, Sobrero et al. , Quarini 2005) , (Farr, Gabelnick et al. 1994) can lead to cervical dysplasia and will usually result in cervical cancer if not caught early and treated. Female barriers are an integral part of protecting a woman's cervix from high-risk strains of HPV (Faundes, Eliast et al. 1994). Despite the existence of a vaccine, in addition there is a simpler, more natural way to protect the cervix. The consistent use of a cervical cap, diaphragm, or condom with every act of intercourse will offer protection against all HPV (Wright, Vessey et al. 1978).

Chlamydia and Gonorrhea are sexually transmitted bacterial infections. Both are treatable and curable, but if they are not detected in the early stages, they can lead to long-term problems such as Pelvic Inflammatory Disease (PID) and infertility. Chlamydia is currently the most common STI in the USA (CDC, 2012) (Marrazzo 2004) (Mar- razzo 2004) (Wright, Vessey et al. 1978). It is especially dangerous as it is often asymptomatic until it reaches advanced stages. Chlamydia can cause damage to the fallopian tubes and can result in infertility. The same is true of gonorrhea. Consistent use of a cervical cap or diaphragm will help to protect the cervix and fallopian tubes from the irreversible damage caused by these dangerous STI's.

An annual exam and Pap smear are essential to a woman's health plan. In the USA, the ACOG recommends that a woman should have her first Pap smear when she turns 21 and have the test repeated every three years as long as the results remain normal, (2017, 2019). The female barrier, while it protects the health of the cervix, must be accompanied by a female or male condom to give all-around protection from STI's. The use of female barriers and male condoms are all-natural forms of contraception and STI prevention that result in no ill side effects for the user.

CHAPTER 16

∾

A BRIGHTER FUTURE

The world is moving toward a more ecological, more sustainable, less disposable, less chemical society. It makes perfect sense that our birth control should follow in the same pattern. It is up to us to promote reform in women's health care. We must spread the message to our health care providers that we want safe, healthy, and affordable contraceptive choices.

I trust that reading my book will be just the beginning of a new and exciting chapter in your quest for natural birth control. I hope all of you who are users will pass this useful information on to those you know and become supporters of the cause yourselves. As an advocate of female barrier birth control, I genuinely believe that informed choices will help lead the way to the revival of cap and diaphragm use.

I look forward to this book creating a stepping- stone to birth control reform. Please visit my Facebook page at Beauty of Natural Birth Control or join my Facebook closed group Beauty of Natural Birth Control Users. You can also email me at beautyofnaturalbirthcontrol@gmail.com.

REFERENCES

(2011). "Multipurpose Prevention Technologies: Biomedical Tools to Prevent HIV-1, HSV-2, and Unintended Pregnancies." <u>Infectious Diseases in Obstetrics and Gynecology</u> **2011**.

(2018). Papanicolaou Smear, StatPearls Publishing, Treasure Island (FL).

ACOG (2017) Pap Smear Resource Overview.

Carslaw, H. and A. Cosh (2016). "Contraception for older women." <u>InnovAiT: Education and inspiration for general practice.</u>

Cervical Barrier Advancement Society. http://www.cervicalbarriers. org/products/methods.cfm

Contraception PHS 933 Lecture 9 Flashcards/Quizlet. https://quizlet. com/109220888/chapter-5-contraception-flash-cards/

de Sanjosé, S., et al. (2019). "Burden of Human Papillomavirus (HPV)-Related Cancers Attributable to HPVs 6/11/16/18/31/33/45/52 and 58." <u>JNCI Cancer Spectrum</u> **2**(4).

Farr, G., et al. (1994). "Contraceptive efficacy and acceptability of the female condom." American Journal of Public Health **84**(12): 1960-1964.

Faundes, A., et al. (1994). "Spermicides and barrier contraception." Current Opinion in Obstetrics and Gynecology **6**(6).

James, T. Contraceptive efficacy. Contraceptive Technology New York, Ardent Media: 779-863.

Koch, J. P. (1982). "The prentif contraceptive cervical cap: Acceptability aspects and their implications for future cap design." Contraception **25**(2): 161-173.

Lehfeldt, H., et al. (1961). "Spermicidal effectiveness of chemical contraceptives used with the firm cervical cap." American Journal of Obstetrics and Gynecology **82**(2): 449-455.

Leitch, W. S. (1986). "Longevity of Ortho Creme (R) and Gynol II (R) in the contraceptive diaphragm." Contraception **34**(4): 381-393.

Linton, A., et al. (2016). "Contraception for the perimenopausal woman." Climacteric **19**(6): 526-534.

Marrazzo, J. M. (2004). "Barriers to infectious disease care among lesbians." Emerging infectious diseases **10**(11): 1974-1978.

Merck (2017) Gardisil 9.

Parenthood, P. (2016). Diaphragm Birth Control | How Safe and Effective is it?

Quarini, C. A. (2005). "History of contraception." Women's Health Medicine 2(5): 28-30.

Roizen, J., et al. (2002). "Oves® contraceptive cap: Short-term acceptability, aspects of use and user satisfaction." Journal of Family Planning and Reproductive Health Care 28(4): 188-192.

Thoreau, H. D. "Quote by Henry David Thoreau: what you Get by Achieving ....".

Vessey, M. and P. Wiggins (1974). "Use-effectiveness of the diaphragm in a selected family planning clinic population in the United Kingdom." Contraception 9(1): 15-21.

Wing, T. A. (2016) Women's Birth Control Choices. Women's Natural Health Practice

Wright, N. H., et al. (1978). "Neoplasia and dysplasia of the cervix uteri and contraception: a possible protective effect of the diaphragm." British Journal of Cancer 38(2): 273-279.

APPENDIX A

~

Female Barrier Fact Sheets

Diaphragm materials and rim styles

The differences between diaphragms are in the materials, silicone or latex, and rim styles: arcing spring, coil spring, and flat spring. The rim style you should use will be determined primarily by your fitter who will make that determination by assessing your vaginal muscle tone and the physical shape of your pelvic anatomy. Diaphragm sizes are standardized in 5 mm increments, and the range of sizes available will vary depending on the maker. Diaphragms from the two of the three significant makers (Ortho and Cooper Surgical) are made of silicone while the Lamberts Reflexions is made of latex.

The advantages of silicone diaphragms are that if properly cared for they should last several times longer than those made of latex and are less likely to contribute to infections. However, silicone diaphragms cost more, don't transmit heat as well as latex and shouldn't be used with silicone lubricants.

The advantages of latex diaphragms are that the thin stretchy dome transmits heat much better than silicone so they feel more natural and they are about half the cost of a silicone diaphragm and they can be used with silicone lubricants. The disadvantages of latex diaphragms are that they can't be used by couples with a latex allergy, they usually need to be replaced sooner than silicone and the porous natural rubber latex if not thoroughly cleaned between wearings is more likely to contribute to infections. Latex diaphragms are also more easily damaged by oily medicines or lubricants than are silicone ones.

Rim Styles:

ARCING SPRING: This rim style has a very sturdy rim with very firm spring strength. Most women are able to use the arcing rim comfortably even women with poor vaginal muscle tone. Arcing spring makers: Ortho All-Flex comes in 4 diameters (65mm to 80mm). It folds in two planes and can be folded anywhere on the rim. Cooper Surgical (Milex) wide seal arcing spring comes in 8 diameter sizes (60mm to 95mm) The Milex Arcing spring folds in only two spots with elbow hinges. Both are made of silicone and both are available in the U.S and Europe.

COIL SPRING: This rim style is intended for women with average vaginal muscle tone and an average pubic notch. It folds into a long flat oval for insertion and can flex in two planes. Coil spring makers are: Cooper Surgical (Milex) wide seal Omniflex and Semina both made of silicone. The Milex Omniflex comes in 8 diameters (60mm to 95mm) and is available in the U.S and Europe. Semina comes in 6 diameters (60mm to 85mm) and is available in South America and Europe. Both the Omniflex and Semina can be folded anywhere on the rim.

FLAT SPRING: The flat spring has a strong rim spring which folds in a single plane into a long flat oval and is intended for women with firm vaginal muscle tone or a shallow pubic notch. Lamberts (Dalston) are the only major maker that still produces latex diaphragms. The Reflexions latex flat spring diaphragm comes in 7 diameters (65mm to 95mm) and is available in the U.S. and Europe. The flat spring diaphragm is the only rim style that can be safely worn on SCUBA dives below 30 feet. That's because the rim will not distort due to water pressure as will the hollow cores of the arcing and coil spring rims.

APPENDIX B

∼

Natural Spermicides

NATURAL SPERMICIDE LABORATORY TEST

April 2009

Time taken to immobilize spermatozoa after contact with spermicides *(average time for ten spermatozoa immobilized 100%)*				
SPERMICIDE			SPERM	
		Level 1	Level 3	Level 5
2% nonoxynol -9	Control	2m 11s	13 m 34s	44m 55s
Lemon, Cornstarch, Honey	NS1	15m 34s	65m 20s	*
Aloe vera, Lemon	NS2	13m 10s	52m 16s	**
Lemon, Salt, Cornstarch	NS3	1m 8s	9m 51s	73m 41s
Manuka honey (UMF 16+)	NS4	9m 4s	19m 42s	138m 3s
Femprotect 3.5% lactic acid	NS5	2m 17s	15m 48s	31m 7s

* sperm still active after 2 hours, all sperm immobile after 4 hours

** still active after 2 hours, all sperm immobile after 3 hours

Method

1). Prepare 6 microscope dimple slides with 1ml of each spermicide controlled at body temp

2). Add 1ml of level 1 semen to one slide at a time straight from the incubator at body temp

3). Time the period for 100% immobilization of 10 sperm in contact at the semen/spermicide junction

4). Average the time taken to immobilize 10 sperm at the spermicide/semen junction

5). Repeat steps 1-4 with level 3 and level 5 semen

6). Compare results to OTC 2.0% nonoxynol-9 spermicide

Please refer to attached sheet for the compounds of each natural spermicide

Semen samples

Three semen samples were obtained from a UK sperm bank. One level 1 (subfertile), one level 3 (average fertile) and one level 5 (super fertile).

Semen parameters for samples used in the test

	Level 2	Level 3	Level 5
pH	6.4	7.1	7.4
Volume (million/ml)	9	35	233
Motility (rapid)	11	25	91
% normal	5	23	72
% abnormal	95	77	28
Anti-sperm antibodies	0	0	0

Results

1). All spermicides immobilized all three levels of sperm quality within the 6-hour post last coitus female barrier minimum removal time

2). NS1 and 2 were less effective than NS3,4,5 at all levels, particularly with level 5 sperm

3). Sperm penetrated the spermicide/semen junction by a maximum of 100microns (one-tenth of a millimeter) with the exception of Manuka honey which did not allow any penetration, suggesting a physical barrier property as well as a spermicidal action

Femprotect - Lactic Acid Contraceptive Gel

Femprotect is a reliable spermicidal gel. NVSH first developed it in the Netherlands for use with diaphragms, cervical caps, and condoms under the name Contracep Green which was tested in the laboratories of NVSH and strictly to the norms of IPPF (International Planned Parenthood Federation). Because of its natural composition, Femprotect doesn't damage latex diaphragms, caps, or condoms. Additionally, Femprotect is a water-based lubricant for use during any sexual activity. (note: Never use oil or petroleum based lubricants together with latex diaphragms, caps or condoms).

Instructions for Use

Diaphragms: Apply 5ml (1tsp) of the gel in the middle of the inside of the dome of the diaphragm. Spread the gel with the help of your finger over the whole inside surface and the inside of the rim.

Cervical Caps: Fill the dome of the cap 1/3 full with gel and follow the instruction for the use of your cap. **Femprotect** is suitable for all kinds of latex cervical caps, Oves cervical caps and Femcaps.

Condoms: Apply a small amount of Femprotect on the penis inside the condom first then a small additional amount on the tip of the outside of the condom before penetration.

Side effects

Femprotect has very few side effects if any. Most women tolerate it well. You can use the gel as long and as often as you like it. In rare cases of reactions, you should stop using Femprotect and ask your healthcare provider or pharmacist for advice. **Femprotect** has no color or odor and does not stain fabric.

Composition (100g tube)

Lactic acid	3.5 %	Sorbic acid	0.1 %
Sodium lactate	4.5 %	Tylose h 300	7.5 %
Glycerol	15.0%	Water	69.4%

Storage

If you keep Femprotect in a cool place (below 35 degrees C), it will last for 12 months (from production date). Please observe the expiration date on the package.

Note

No method of contraception is 100% effective; therefore, decisions made about your contraception should be informed and carefully considered. Natural spermicides have been shown to compare favorably to chemical spermicides in immobilizing sperm in laboratory tests and anecdotally with similar efficacy when used with a diaphragm or cap. However; because there have been no large-scale clinical trials to prove the efficacy of natural spermicides, using these as an alternative to chemical spermicides has to be an individual woman's informed choice.

Natural Spermicide Recipes

Homemade spermicide – UK/Europe formulation

- 1 TBS (18ml) pure Aloe Vera
- 4 drops lemon juice

Mix well and store in the refrigerator for up to two weeks or in the freezer for up to six months

Homemade spermicide – U.S formulation

- 1 TBS (15ml) pure Aloe Vera
- 3 drops lemon juice

Mix well and store in the refrigerator for up to two weeks or in the freezer for up to six months

Honey

Manuka Honey at UMF 16+ Lemon, Honey, Cornstarch
- Lemon juice (14 drops)
- Honey
- Cornstarch (tsp.)

Lactic Acid Gel

It has a neutral smell & natural sensation and keeps for about five months if kept in an airtight container or tube. This recipe should make approximately 100g of gel:
- 8 g Amylum Tritici (wheat starch)
- 11 g Aqua purificata (distilled water)
- 3.5 g Acidum lacticum (lactic acid)

- 76 g Glycerinum (85%)
- 4 g Tragacantha albissim; pulverized
- 10 g Spiritus (90%)

Allow 8g wheat starch to soak for at least 15 minutes in 11 g distilled water in which 1 g lactic acid has been dissolved. Stir several times. Afterward, add 76 g Glycerinum and mix well. In a different receptacle, mix 4g Tragacantha with 10 g Spiritus, stir thoroughly and add this mixture to the first mixture. Then, heat the combined mixture in a boiling bain-marie and stir continuously until all alcohol has vaporized completely (check by smelling!) and the gel has thickened and become viscous (approximately 20-40 min.). During this process and at the end, add water several times to supplement the vaporized share to make 100 g.

APPENDIX C

~

Female Barrier Effectiveness

Method	Perfect Use	Typical Use
Effectiveness Comparison of User-Directed Contraceptive Methods		
Oral Contraceptives	99%	92%
CycleBeads/SDM	95%	88%
Male Condom	98%	85%
Diaphragm	94%	84%
Spermicide	82%	71%
No Method	15%	15%

Source: Adapted from *Contraceptive Technology*, 18th edition.

Statistics for Dual Protection

Cervical Barriers (Diaphragm)

94% effective alone with perfect use - 86% effective alone with typical use

Cervical Barriers + The Contraceptive Implant = 99.99% effective with perfect use - 99.98% effective with typical use

Cervical Barriers + Intrauterine Devices = 99.99% effective with perfect use - 99.89% effective with typical use

Cervical Barriers + Depo-Provera = 99.98% effective perfect use - 99.58% typical use

Cervical Barriers + Combination OCP ("*The Pill*") = 99.98% effective with perfect use - 98.88% effective with typical use

Cervical Barriers + The Contraceptive Patch = 99.98% effective with perfect use - 98.88% effective with typical use

Cervical Barriers + Minipills = 99.98% effective with perfect use - 98.6% effective with typical use

Cervical Barriers + Male Condoms = 99.88% effective perfect use - 97.9% effective with typical use

Cervical Barriers + Fertility Awareness = 99.88% effective with perfect use - 97.2% effective with typical use

Cervical Barriers + Female Condoms = 99.7% effective with perfect use - 97% effective with typical use

Cervical Barriers + *Emergency Contraception* = 99.34% effective with perfect use - 96.5% effective with typical use

Cervical Barriers + Withdrawal = 99.76% effective with perfect use - 96.22% effective with typical use

Spermicides with cervical barriers are not listed because spermicide is supposed to be used with them, so effectiveness rates for barrier methods already include the addition of a spermicide. Since the sponge already contains a spermicide, spermicide was also excluded from combination with the sponge.

95% effective with perfect use - 79% effective with typical use
Female Condoms + The Contraceptive Implant = 99.99% effective with perfect use - 99.97% effective with typical use

Female Condoms + Intrauterine Devices = 99.99% effective with perfect use - 99.37% effective with typical use

Female Condoms + Depo-Provera = 99.99% effective with perfect use - 99.37% effective with typical use

Female Condoms + Combination OCP = 99.98% effective with perfect use - 98.32% effective with typical use

Female Condoms + The Contraceptive Patch = 99.98% effective with perfect use - 98.32% effective with typical use

Female Condoms + the Vaginal Ring = 99.98% effective with perfect use - 98.32% effective with typical use

Female Condoms + Minipills = 99.98% effective with perfect use - 97.9% effective with typical use

Female Condoms + Cervical Barriers = 99.7% effective with perfect use - 97% effective with typical use

Female Condoms + the Sponge = 99.55% effective with perfect use - 96.64% effective with typical use

Female Condoms + Fertility Awareness = 99.9% effective with perfect use - 95.8% effective with typical use

Female Condoms + Emergency Contraception = 99.45% effective with perfect use - 94.75% effective with typical use

Female Condoms + Withdrawal = 99.8% effective with perfect use - 94.33% effective with typical use

Female Condoms + Spermicide = 99.1% effective with perfect use - 93.91% effective with typical use

Don't forget! *The addition of condoms to any method **always** carries the joint benefit of both allowing men a part in birth control and greatly reducing the risks of sexually transmitted infections.*

APPENDIX D

~

History of Birth Control

Women and men have long tried many methods to prevent pregnancy. Prior to modern methods of birth control, women relied on withdrawal or periodic abstinence. These methods often failed.

Around 3000 B.C. Condoms made from such materials as fish bladders, linen sheaths, and animal intestines.

Around 1500 First spermicides introduced which used condoms made from linen cloth sheaths and soaked in a chemical solution and dried before using.

1838 Condoms and diaphragms made from vulcanized rubber.

1873 The Comstock Act passed in the United States prohibiting advertisements, information, and distribution of birth control and allowing the postal service to confiscate birth control sold through the mail.

1916 Margaret Sanger opens first birth control clinic in the United States. The next year she was deemed guilty of maintaining a public nuisance and sentenced to jail for 30 days. Once released, she re-opened her clinic and continued to persevere through more arrests and prosecutions.

1938 In a case involving Margaret Sanger, a judge lifted the federal ban on birth control, ending the Comstock era. Diaphragms, also known as womb veils, became a popular method of birth control.

1950 While in her 80s, Sanger underwrote the research necessary to create the first human birth control pill. She raised $150,000 for the project.

1960 The first oral contraceptive, Enovid, was approved by the US Food and Drug Administration (FDA) as contraception.

1965 The Supreme Court (in Griswold v. Connecticut) gave married couples the right to use birth control, ruling that it was protected in the Constitution as a right to privacy. However, millions of unmarried women in 26 states were still denied birth control.

1968 FDA approved intrauterine devices (IUDs), bringing early versions like the Lippes Loop and Copper 7 to market.

1970 Feminists challenged the safety of oral contraceptives (the Pill) at well-publicized Congressional hearings. As a result, the formulation of the Pill was changed, and the package insert for prescription drugs came into being.

1972 The Supreme Court (in Baird v. Eisenstadt) legalized birth control for all citizens of this country, irrespective of marital status.

1974 The FDA suspended sale of the Dalkon Shield IUD due to infections and seven documented deaths among users. Although other IUD designs were not implicated, most IUDs were slowly taken off the US market due to the escalating costs of lawsuits in subsequent years.

1980s Pills with low doses of hormones were introduced, along with a new copper IUD, ParaGard (1998). (CuT380a). Growing awareness of the Yuzpe regimen for emergency contraception.

1990s Introduction of Norplant, the first contraceptive implant (1990),DepoProvera, an injectable method (1992), FC1/Reality, a female condom (1993) and Plan B, and a dedicated emergency contraceptive product (1999).

2000s Rapid expansion in method availability and improvements in safety and effectiveness, including introduction of Mirena, a new levonorgestrel-releasing IUD (2000), Ortho Evra, a hormonal patch (2001), Nuvaring, a vaginal ring (2001), Essure, a method of transcervical female sterilization (2002), Implanon, a single-rod implant (2006), and FC2, an improved female condom (2009).

2002 The first implant, Norplant, is taken off the US market.

2010s Ella, a new emergency contraceptive pill (2010) and Skyla, a new levonorgestrel-releasing IUD (2013) are introduced. Growing use of the copper IUD for emergency contraception.

2013 After protracted regulatory and legal battles, one brand of emergency contraceptive pill (Plan B One-Step) becomes available without a prescription on drug store shelves.

Today More research is needed on woman-controlled methods that protect against STIs and birth control for men. Barriers to accessing reliable contraception remain for women worldwide.

Excerpt from the 2011 edition of Our Bodies, Ourselves: https://www.ourbodiesourselves.org/publications/our-bodies-ourselves-2011/

APPENDIX E

∽

Picture Library

Cervical Caps

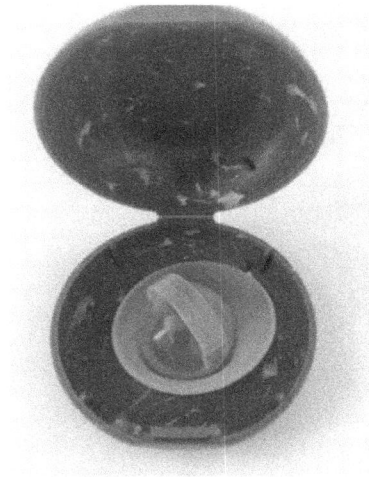

FemCap

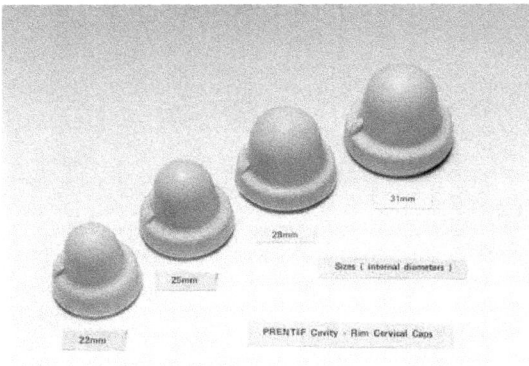

Range of Prentif Caps

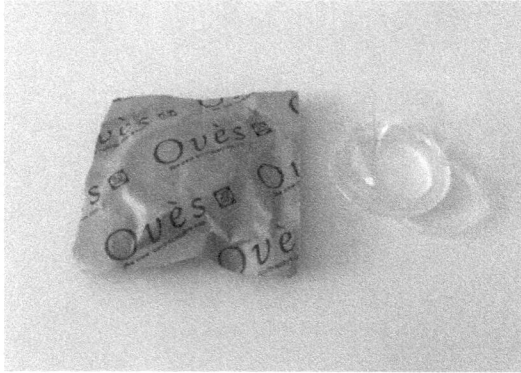

Oves

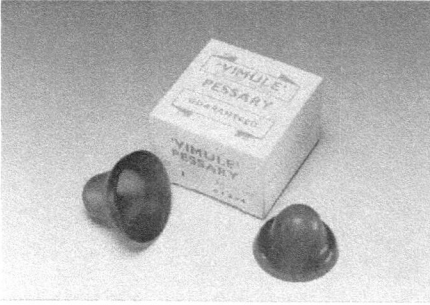

Natural Latex Vimule Cap

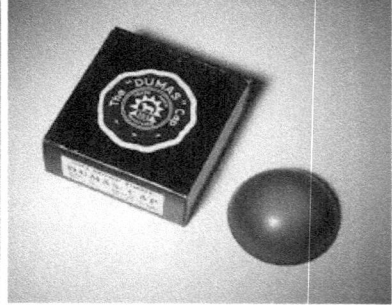

Natural Latex Dumas Cap

Modern Diaphragms

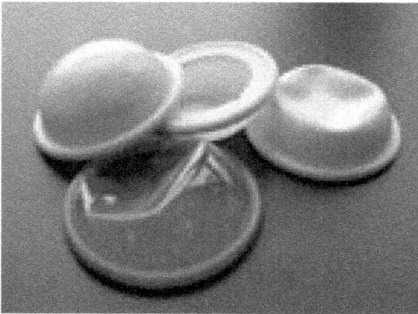

Ortho Coil, Milex Omniflex, Milex Arcing, Semina

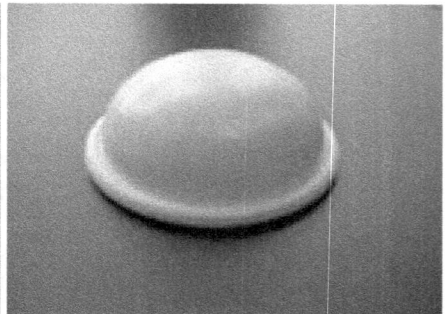

Ortho Coil

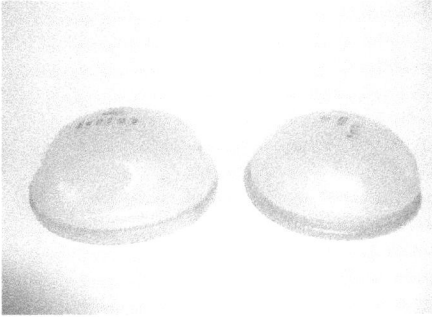

Menstrual Diaphragms

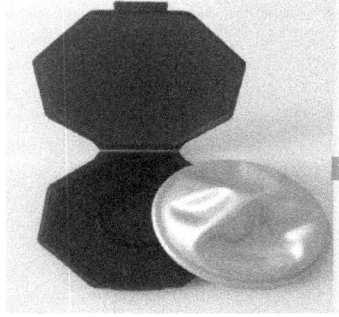

Reflexions

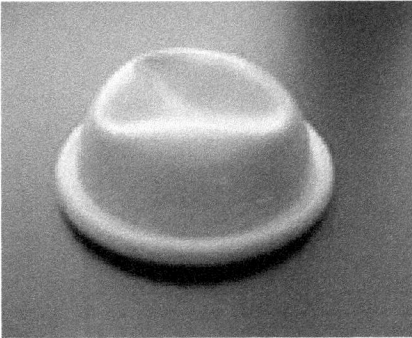

Ortho All-Flex

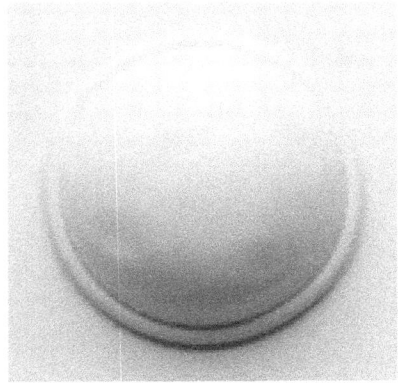

Ortho White

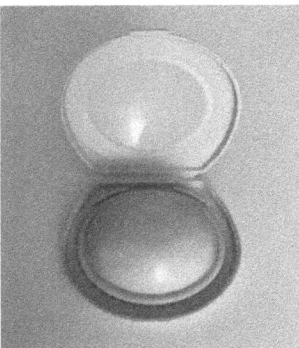

Milex Arcing

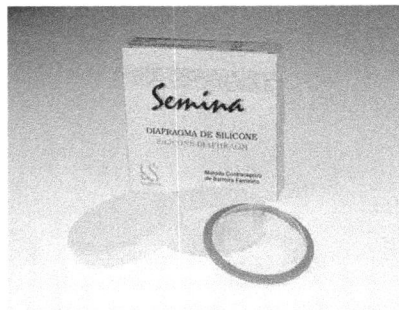

Semina

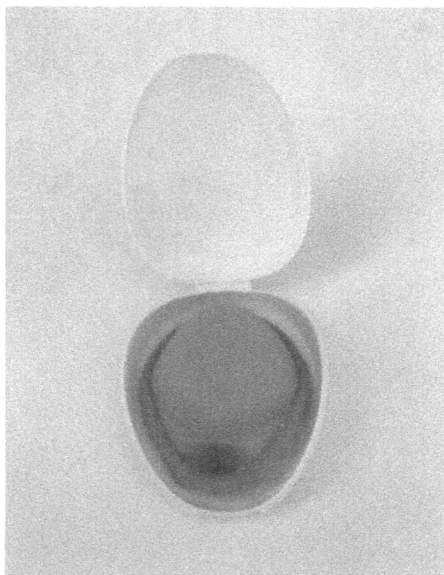

Caya

Vintage Diaphragms

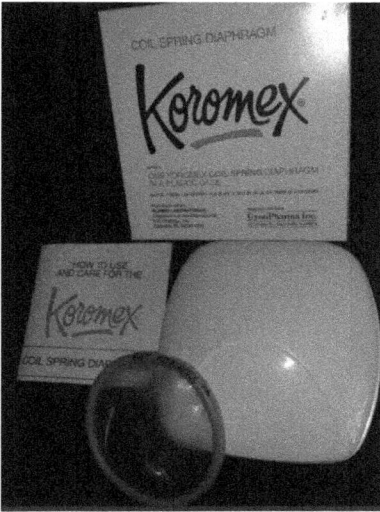

Koromex Coil Spring

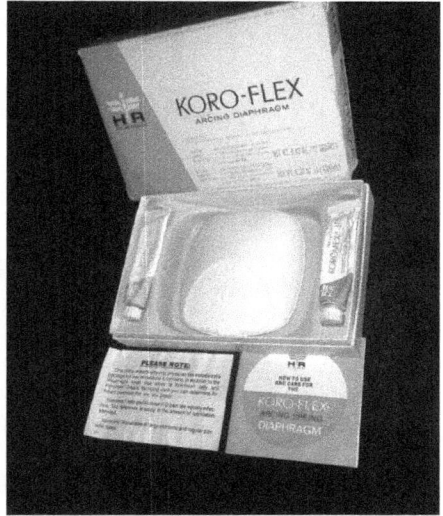

Koromex Arcing Spring

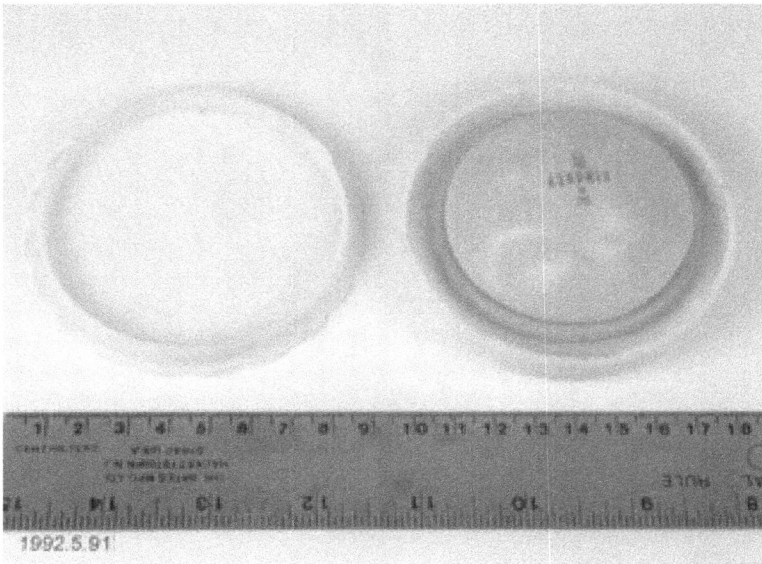

Koromex

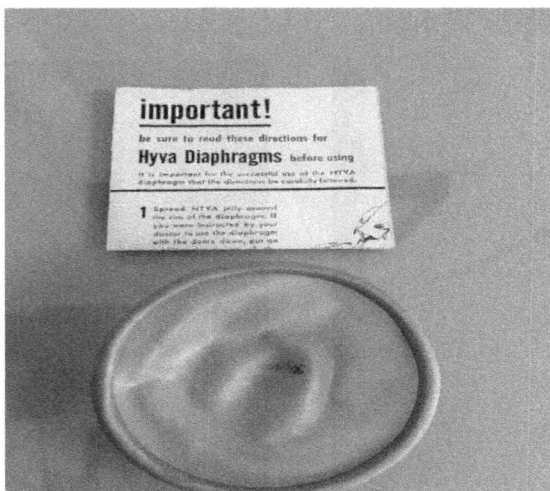

Huya

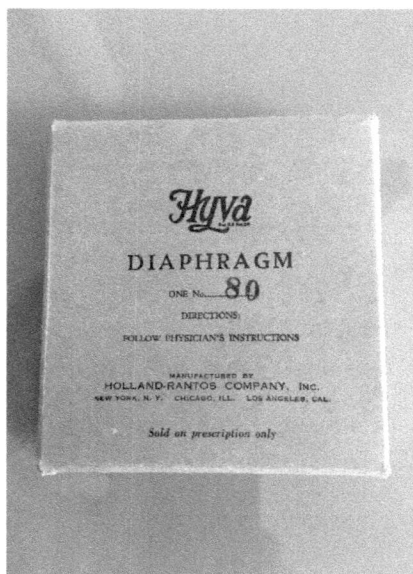

Huya

www.ingramcontent.com/pod-product-compliance
Lightning Source LLC
Chambersburg PA
CBHW032118280326
41933CB00009B/898